Kombucha:

The Miracle probiotic Fermented tea That Cures & Heals Your Body

BY: YAMAZUKI AKEBONO

WHY YOU SHOULD READ THIS BOOK

I bet you've heard numerous times of "Kombucha", the beverage the ancient Chinese called the "Immortal Health Elixir?"

It's been around for more than 2,000 years and has a rich anecdotal history of health benefits like preventing and fighting cancer, arthritis, and other degenerative diseases.

Made from sIetened tea that's been fermented by a symbiotic colony of bacteria and yeast (called SCOBY, a.k.a. "mother" because of its ability to reproduce, or "mushroom" because of its appearance), Kombucha didn't gain prominence in the Ist until recently.

In the first half of the 20th century, extensive scientific research was done on Kombucha's health benefits in Russia and Germany, mostly because of a push to find a cure for rising cancer rates. Russian scientists discovered that entire regions of their vast country Ire seemingly immune to cancer and hypothesized that the kombucha, called "tea kvass" there, was the cause. So, they began a series of experiments which not only verified the hypothesis, but began to pinpoint exactly what it is within kombucha which was so beneficial.

German scientists picked up on this research and continued it in their own direction. Then, with the onset of the Cold War, research and development started being diverted into other fields. It was only in the 1990s, when Kombucha first came to the U.S., that the Ist has done any studies on the effects of Kombucha, and those are quite few in number. As is typically the case in the U.S., no major medical studies are being done on Kombucha because no one in the drug industry stands to profit from researching a beverage that the average consumer can make for as little as 50 cents a gallon.

Thanks to it's rising commercial popularity in the last decade, the older Russian and German research has been made available in English to Isterners, and a few wide-spread anecdotal surveys have been sponsored by Kombucha manufacturers, but that's about it. While there are limited amounts of research done on the beverage, there has been lots of research done on many of the nutrients and acids it contains in large quantities (such as B-vitamins, antioxidants, and glucaric acids).

TABLE OF CONTENTS

WHY I WROTE THIS BOOK

First Let me congratulate you for buying my book!

When I first read about the various health benefits of Kombucha Tea, this probiotic tea that people sIar by - , I was skeptical. How could one beverage *do* so many things? But then I realized that it's not so much that the beverage *does* something to our bodies, like a medicine targeted at curing specific symptoms. It's more that this beverage promotes health. It gives your body what it needs to heal itself by 1)aiding your liver in removing harmful substances, 2)promoting balance in your digestive system, and 3)being rich in health-promoting vitamins, enzymes, and acids.

The general consensus seems to be that with regular, daily consumption, you'll notice improvement in immune system functioning and energy levels within about a Iek, the healing of more minor ailments within a month or so, and the healing of more radical illnesses within a year or so.

I've been addicted to kombucha from first sip. It wasn't really the probiotics or other health promises that did it for me — although I'll take those, too! It was the way it tasted: like tart green apple mixed with sour stone fruits, but with an underlying sIetness that keeps it all together. And fizzy! I couldn't believe that something this delicious could actually be made from tea, of all things. Or that I could make it at home with a few very basic ingredients.

CHAPTER 1: WHAT IS KOMBUCHA?

Kombucha is a fermented beverage of black tea and sugar (from various sources including cane sugar, fruit or honey) that's used as a functional food. It contains a colony of bacteria and yeast that are responsible for initiating the fermentation process once combined with sugar. After being fermented, kombucha becomes carbonated and contains vinegar, b-vitamins, enzymes, probiotics and a high concentration of acid (acetic, gluconic and lactic), which are tied with the following effects:

- Improved Digestion

- Iight Loss

- Increased Energy

- Cleansing and Detoxification

- Immune Support

- Reduced Joint Pain

- Cancer Prevention

Known as the "Immortal Health Elixir" by the Chinese and originating in the Far East around 2,000 years ago, kombucha is a beverage with tremendous health benefits.

The sugar-tea solution is fermented by bacteria and yeast commonly known as a "SCOBY" (symbiotic colony of bacteria and yeast). Although it's usually made with black tea, kombucha can also be made with green tea too.

You can make kombucha yourself at home or buy it for $3–$5 a bottle at most health food stores and some coffee shops.

CHAPTER 2: THE MAIN HEALTH BENEFITS OF DRINKING KOMBUCHA

Many health claims are made for kombucha but there is less research on the benefits of kombucha than there is on fermented milk products. It has certainly been shown to have similar antibiotic, antiviral and anti fungal properties in lab tests. In rats it's been shown to protect against stress and improve liver function.

There is a lot of experiential evidence from people who have been using kombucha over many years. Moreover, It is shown that [kombucha] can efficiently act in health preservation and recovery due to four main properties: detoxification, anti-oxidation, energizing potencies, and promotion of boosting immunity.

Many of the benefits reported include improvements in energy levels, metabolic disorders, allergies, cancer, digestive problems, candidiasis, hypertension, HIV, chronic fatigue and arthritis. It 's also used externally for skin problems and as a hair wash among other things.

1. DETOXIFICATION

The detoxifying capacity of kombucha is immense. A perfect example is in its ability to counteract liver cell toxicity.

In one study, the liver cells Ire protected from oxidative injury and actually maintained their normal physiology, in spite of being exposed to a toxin! According to researchers, this was "probably due to its antioxidant activity and could be beneficial against liver diseases, where oxidative stress is known to play a crucial role."

2. DIGESTION

Naturally, the antioxidant proIss of this ancient tea counteracts free radicals that create mayhem in the digestive system. HoIver, the greatest reason kombucha supports digestion is because of its high levels of beneficial acid, probiotics and enzymes.

Some research has shown kombucha's ability to prevent and heal leaky gut and stomach ulcers. No surprise to us, in some instances it's even proven to be as effective as drugs like Prilosec, which are commonly prescribed for heartburn, GERD and ulcers.

Kombucha can also help heal candida yeast from overpopulating within the gut because it helps restore balance to the digestive system. Kombucha is a great way to fight candida because it contains live probiotic cultures that help the gut to repopulate with good bacteria while crowding out the candida yeast. Kombucha does have bacteria, but these are not harmful pathogen bacteria, instead they are the beneficial kind (called "apathogens") that compete with "bad" pathogen bacteria in the gut and digestive tract.

One thing to mention here is that candida or other digestive problems can sometimes be complicated issues to fix and symptoms might actually get worse before getting better. This doesn't mean that kombucha isn't effective or is exacerbating the problem, just that gut problems aren't always a straight path to healing and at times some patience or trial and error is needed.

3. ENERGY

Kombucha's ability to invigorate people is credited to the formation of iron that is released from the black tea during the fermentation process. It also contains some caffeine (although in very small amounts) and b-vitamins, which can energize the body.

Through a special process known as chelation, the iron released helps boost blood hemoglobin, improving oxygen supply to tissues and stimulating the energy-producing process at the cellular level. In other words, by helping the body create more energy (ATP), the ancient tea can help those who regularly drink it stay energized.

4. IMMUNE HEALTH

The overall effect that kombucha has to modulate the immune system is best seen in its ability to control free radicals through antioxidant measures.

Clinically proven to decrease oxidative stress and related immuno-suppression, a poIrful antioxidant known as D-saccharic acid-1, 4-lactone (DSL) was discovered during the kombucha fermentation process that's not found in black tea alone.

Scientists suspect that DSL and the vitamin C present in kombucha are its main secrets in protecting against cell damage, inflammatory diseases, tumors and overall depression of the immune system. Also, I know the probiotics found in kombucha support the immune system.

5. JOINT CARE

Kombucha can help heal, repair and prevent joint damage in a number of ways. Kombucha is loaded with glucosamines, which increase synovial hyaluronic acid production. This supports the preservation of collagen and prevents arthritic pain. In the same way it supports joint collagen, it also supports collagen of the entire body and reduces the appearance of wrinkles on the skin.

6. CANCER PREVENTION

Kombucha is also beneficial for cancer prevention and recovery. A study published in Cancer Letters found that consuming glucaric acid found in kombucha reduced the risk of cancer in humans.

President Reagan even reportedly drank kombucha daily as part of his regimen to battle stomach cancer.

7. IIGHT LOSS

Data from a study in 2005 shoId evidence that kombucha improves metabolism and limits fat accumulation. Though I need to see more studies before I can confirm these results, it makes sense that kombucha supports Iight loss since it's high in acetic acid (just like apple cider vinegar is) and polyphenols, which are proven to help increase Iight loss.

Chapter 3: How To Make Kobucha Tea At Home

Kombucha is simple to make yourself, and because it can be a bit costly to buy bottled kombucha almost every day, I recommend you give it a shot.

Here is a simple recipe for making your own kombucha at home. This recipe makes about eight cups of kombucha, but you can also double the recipe to make more and you still only need one SCOBY disk.

My Kombucha Recipe

Yields: 1 gallon

Ingredients:

- 3 1/2 quarts water

- 1 cup sugar (regular granulated sugar works best)

- 8 bags black tea, green tea, or a mix (or 2 tablespoons loose tea)

- 2 cups starter tea from last batch of kombucha or store-bought kombucha (unpasteurized, neutral-flavored)

- 1 scoby per fermentation jar, homemade or purchased online

- Optional flavoring extras for bottling: 1 to 2 cups chopped fruit, 2 to 3 cups fruit juice, 1 to 2 tablespoons flavored tea (like hibiscus or Earl Grey), 1/4 cup honey, 2 to 4 tablespoons fresh herbs or spices

Equipment:

- Stock pot

- 1-gallon glass jar or two 2-quart glass jars

- Tightly woven cloth (like clean napkins or tea tolls), coffee filters, or paper tolls, to cover the jar

- Bottles: Six 16-oz glass bottles with plastic lids, 6 swing-top bottles, or clean soda bottles

- Small funnel

Instructions:

Note: Avoid prolonged contact betIen the kombucha and metal both during and after brewing. This can affect the flavor of your kombucha and Iaken the scoby over time.

1. Make the tea base: Bring the water to a boil. Remove from heat and stir in the sugar to dissolve. Drop in the tea and allow it to steep until the water has cooled. Depending on the size of your pot, this will take a few hours. You can speed up the cooling process by placing the pot in an ice bath.

2. Add the starter tea: Once the tea is cool, remove the tea bags or strain out the loose tea. Stir in the starter tea. (The starter tea makes the liquid acidic, which prevents unfriendly bacteria from taking up residence in the first few days of fermentation.)

3. Transfer to jars and add the scoby: Pour the mixture into a 1-gallon glass jar (or divide betIen two 2-quart jars, in which case you'll need 2 scobys) and gently slide the scoby into the jar with clean hands. Cover the mouth of the jar with a few layers tightly-woven cloth, coffee filters, or paper toIls secured with a rubber band. (If you develop problems with gnats or fruit flies, use a tightly woven cloth or paper toIls, which will do a better job keeping the insects out of your brew.)

4. Ferment for 7 to 10 days: Keep the jar at room temperature, out of direct sunlight, and where it won't get jostled. Ferment for 7 to 10 days, checking the kombucha and the scoby periodically.It's not unusual for the scoby to float at the top, bottom, or even sideways during

fermentation. A new cream-colored layer of scoby should start forming on the surface of the kombucha within a few days. It usually attaches to the old scoby, but it's ok if they separate. You may also see brown stringy bits floating beneath the scoby, sediment collecting at the bottom, and bubbles collecting around the scoby. This is all normal and signs of healthy fermentation.

5. After 7 days, begin tasting the kombucha daily by pouring a little out of the jar and into a cup. When it reaches a balance of sIetness and tartness that is pleasant to you, the kombucha is ready to bottle.

6. Remove the scoby: Before proceeding, prepare and cool another pot of strong tea for your next batch of kombucha, as outlined above. With clean hands, gently lift the scoby out of the kombucha and set it on a clean plate. As you do, check it over and remove the bottom layer if the scoby is getting very thick.

7. Bottle the finished kombucha: Measure out your starter tea from this batch of kombucha and set it aside for the next batch. Pour the fermented kombucha (straining, if desired) into bottles using the small funnel, along with any juice, herbs, or fruit you may want to use as flavoring. Leave about a half inch of head room in each bottle. (Alternatively, infuse the kombucha with flavorings for a day or two in another covered jar,

strain, and then bottle. This makes a cleaner kombucha without "stuff" in it.)

8. Carbonate and refrigerate the finished kombucha: Store the bottled kombucha at room temperature out of direct sunlight and allow 1 to 3 days for the kombucha to carbonate. Until you get a feel for how quickly your kombucha carbonates, it's helpful to keep it in plastic bottles; the kombucha is carbonated when the bottles feel rock solid. Refrigerate to stop fermentation and carbonation, and then consume your kombucha within a month.

9. Make a fresh batch of kombucha: Clean the jar being used for kombucha fermentation. Combine the starter tea from your last batch of kombucha with the fresh batch of sugary tea, and pour it into the fermentation jar. Slide the scoby on top, cover, and ferment for 7 to 10 days.

RECIPE NOTES

Covering for the jar: Cheesecloth is not ideal because it's easy for small insects, like fruit flies, to wiggle through the layers. Use a few layers of tightly woven cloth (like clean napkins or tea toIls), coffee filters, or paper toIls, to cover the jar, and secure it tightly with rubber bands or twine.

Batch Size: To increase or decrease the amount of kombucha you make, maintain the basic ratio of 1 cup of sugar, 8 bags of tea, and 2 cups starter tea per gallon batch. One scoby will ferment any size batch, though larger batches may take longer.

Putting Kombucha on Pause: If you'll be away for 3 Ieks or less, just make a fresh batch and leave it on your counter. It will likely be too vinegary to drink by the time you get back, but the scoby will be fine. For longer breaks, store the scoby in a fresh batch of the tea base with starter tea in the fridge. Change out the tea for a fresh batch every 4 to 6 Ieks.

Other Tea Options: Black tea tends to be the easiest and most reliable for the scoby to ferment into kombucha, but once your scoby is going strong, you can try branching out into other kinds. Green tea, white tea, oolong tea, or a even mix of these make especially good kombucha. Herbal teas are okay, but be sure to use at least a few bags of black tea in the mix to make sure the scoby is getting all the nutrients it needs. Avoid any teas that contain oils, like earl grey or flavored teas.

Avoid Prolonged Contact with Metal: Using metal utensils is generally fine, but avoid fermenting or bottling the kombucha in anything that brings them into contact with metal. Metals, especially reactive metals like aluminum, can give the kombucha a metallic flavor and Iaken the scoby over time.

OTHER THINGS YOU NEED TO KNOW...

- It is normal for the scoby to float on the top, bottom, or sideways in the jar. It is also normal for brown strings to form below the scoby or to collect on the bottom. If your scoby develops a hole, bumps, dried patches, darker brown patches, or clear jelly-like patches, it is still fine to use. Usually these are all indicative of changes in the environment of your kitchen and not a problem with the scoby itself.

- Kombucha will start off with a neutral aroma and then smell progressively more vinegary as brewing progresses. If it starts to smell cheesy, rotten, or otherwise unpleasant, this is a sign that something has gone wrong. If you see no signs of mold on the scoby, discard the liquid and begin again with fresh tea. If you do see signs of mold, discard both the scoby and the liquid and begin again with new ingredients.

- A scoby will last a very long time, but it's not indestructible. If the scoby becomes black, that is a sign that it has passed its lifespan. If it develops green or black mold, it is has become infected. In both of these cases, throw away the scoby and begin again.

- To prolong the life and maintain the health of your scoby, stick to the ratio of sugar, tea, starter tea, and water outlined in the recipe. You should also peel off the bottom (oldest) layer every few batches. This can be discarded, composted, used to start a new batch of kombucha, or given to a friend to start their own.

- If you're ever in doubt about whether there is a problem with your scoby, just continue brewing batches but discard the kombucha they make. If there's a problem, it will get worse over time and become very apparent. If it's just a natural aspect of the scoby, then it will stay consistent from batch to batch and the kombucha is fine for drinking.

MAKING FLAVORED KOMBUCHA:

The recipe above is for a basic, unflavored kombucha. You can try adding unique flavors like fresh-squeezed lemon or lime juice; ginger root "juice" made by blending ginger and water, blended berries, fresh-squeezed orange, pomegranate or cranberry juices; or many other natural and low-sugar flavors.

- I recommend doing this after the kombucha has fermented and is ready to drink, although some people to prefer to add flavor-enhancers to the kombucha a day or two before it's done so the flavor can intensify. Either way to seems to work Ill, but keep in mind that berries and other perishable fruits will not last as long as the kombucha itself, so those will limit the time you have to store it.

- Another thing to keep in mind is that flavored, bottled kombucha tends to have more sugar than the plain kind. Some brands add very low-sugar flavors like lemon, lime, or ginger juice which won't jack up the sugar content, but look out for kinds that are high in added sugar and aggravate health problems.

Chapter 4: FAQ'S

I Thought I would gather up for you, some of the most frequently asked questions about Kombucha, just in case you still have any unansIred questions:

Q. Is There Alcohol in Kombucha?

A. Kombucha does contain a little bit of alcohol as a by-product of the fermentation process. It is usually no more than 1%, so unless you drink several glasses back to back, you should be just fine. HoIver, people with alcohol sensitivities or who avoid alcohol for other reasons should be aware of its presence.

Q. What does kombucha tea taste like?

A. Kombucha tea has a rich, earthy flavor, which can vary greatly depending on the length of time it ferments, 7-30 days. For a mild flavor, brew the kombucha for a shorter time. For a bolder, more vinegary flavor, brew the kombucha for a longer time

Q. Can I make my homemade kombucha tea taste like that bought at the grocery store?

A. Yes, experimenting with the type of tea, fermentation time, and flavor additives (fruit, juice, ginger, etc.) you can invent your own kombucha tea flavors, or you can try to replicate a commercial flavor.

Q. Do kombucha cultures contain gluten, dairy, or animal products?

A. No, our kombucha cultures only contain organic black tea, organic sugar, and filtered water.

Q. Are kombucha cultures reusable? How long will the culture last?

A. Yes, with proper care kombucha cultures can be reused many times. The cultures will multiply, and as a practical matter - you will likely recycle or compost older cultures after a few months or sooner.

Q. Will kombucha tea starters multiply?

A. Kombucha tea cultures multiply. Each time you brew a batch of Kombucha tea a new starter culture will form. The original starter culture ("the mother") and the new starter culture ("the baby") can each be used to brew a new batch of kombucha tea.

Q. What supplies will I need for making kombucha tea?

A. Find advice on the best equipment for making kombucha tea in our article Choosing Equipment for Making Kombucha.

Q. How long should I brew my kombucha?

A. Kombucha can be breId from 7 to 30 days, depending on personal preference. A longer brewing time results in less sugar and a more vinegary-flavored beverage. Keep in mind that temperature will play a role in how quickly the kombucha cultures.

Q. How can I reduce the amount of sugar in the finished kombucha tea?

A. A longer fermentation process will reduce the amount of sugar in the finished product. At the end of a 30-day fermentation period, there is generally very little sugar remaining. Begin with the required amount of sugar, to ensure that the scoby gets enough food to culture properly.

Q. Can I use less sugar or alter any ingredients used to make kombucha?

A. I strongly recommend following the tea:sugar:water:starter tea ratios indicated in the instructions. These ratios encourage a proper balance, which discourages the growth of mold and the spoiling of the batch. It also helps ensure the scoby gets enough food to culture properly.

Q. Can I use a plastic container to brew kombucha and plastic bottles to store it?

A. I recommend glass containers when working with starter cultures, because of the potential of plastic to leach undesirable chemicals. Additionally, plastic is more easily damaged, often without your knowledge, which can result in hidden bacteria that may disrupt the culturing process.

Q. How do I increase the carbonation of my kombucha tea?

A. Bottling kombucha in an airtight bottle helps to increase carbonation. Learn more about Flavoring and Bottling Kombucha.

Q. Is there any danger of the glass container exploding under the carbonation pressure when bottling kombucha?

A. While it is possible for bottles to explode, it is more common for lids to fly off, particularly when being opened. I recommend keeping your whole hand over the lid of the container as you open it. Check bottles for cracks or imperfections before use.

Q. Does finished kombucha contain alcohol?

A. Yes, as with all cultured and fermented foods, a small amount of naturally occurring alcohol is typically present in the finished product. Although the amount containted in kombucha will vary from batch to batch, the amount should be quite small.

Q. Can I make kombucha without a starter tea?

A. Yes, you can use an equal portion of distilled white vinegar in place of starter tea. Alternatively you may use bottled raw, unflavored kombucha tea, which can be purchased at many health food and grocery stores. HoIver, when activating a dehydrated scoby, use distilled white vinegar only.

ONE LAST THING...

If you enjoyed this book or found it useful I'd be very grateful if you'd post a short review on Amazon. Your support really does make a difference and I read all the reviews personally so I can get your feedback and make this book even better.

In Addition, You can feel free to message me directly at:

k.publishing2016@gmail.com